LIVING

FROM OUR

GARDEN

MEDITERRANEAN STYLE

Dick Handscombe

Living Well from Our Garden - Mediterranean Style

First edition published September 2011
This revised edition published May 2013

Design by Kevin Turnbull.

Author photograph by Clodagh Brown.

Illustrations by author.

Diagram art work page 6 Lynne Godfrey www.jigsawdesign.biz

Self published by author using Amazon Create Space

ISBN: 978-1484873632
        1484873637

This book is based on what the author has done, does do and intends to do to improve the holistic quality of the health and lives of himself and his wife through their holistic garden, the diversity of ecological foods and drinks they produce harvest and consume on a daily basis and the environment in which they live. There is no guarantee that their practices will do the same for you. It may be wise, especially if taking a course of medications, to discuss any significant changes in practices with your medical advisor before you take action.

CONTENTS

Page

Acknowledgements

The support and long term effort put in by my wife Clodagh to the development and maintenance of our holistic garden, allotment and olive grove is much appreciated.

The timely publication of this book would not have been possible without the long term support of many friends with converging interests, who helped make our self sufficient adventure a success. There are too many to list so Spanish wise thanks to all with an abrazo.

Many thanks to Kevin Turnbull and Jesus Poveda Mataix of Vilsor Impresores for their enthusiastic acceptance and achievement of a tight deadline for the design and printing of the first version of this book and likewise to Amazon Create Space for this version.

Dedications

To those that wish to live well, perhaps very well, from their own self sufficient efforts in their Mediterranean Gardens worldwide whether a large plot around a villa, a rough patch of land around a rural home, or a container garden high up in an apartment block.

Also in memory of those members of the human race who from 27,000 years BC lived before me in the La Drova valley evolving an understanding of the potential wellness of plants and animals, and the healthiest ways to grow harvest eat or drink them. That is until the new human led construction, chemical and medical professions came to believe that they could replace nature, or at least make more money by so doing. It took almost 30,000 years to develop the agriculture of the valley and only 30 to almost destroy it.

Last but firstly, fond memories to my long deceased father and grandfather who first stimulated me to be interested in gardening and cooking, and to gain related scout badges in the 1940's.

Authors Introduction

Living Well from Our Mediterranean Garden is a natural follow on from the following quartet of earlier books Your Garden in Spain, Apartment Gardening Mediterranean Style, Growing Healthy Fruit in Spain and Growing Healthy Vegetables in Spain.

The book explores how to live well from a Mediterranean garden in terms of healthily, gastronomically and economically. It has been a long time in gestation since my wife Clodagh and I gave a talk to a Costa Blanca Spain U3A conference with the same title, but a busy life style restricts writing time. However, the current wide spread health gastronomic and economic strife at individual, family and national levels suggests that it is now timely to publish. The book is based on our wide ranging experiences and experiments in achieving a high level of self sufficiency and a low cost approach to holistic wellness from our gardening efforts since we came to Spain 25 years ago, and in particular after I retired early following cancer operations in 1993. In that time four dry abandoned agricultural terraces have become peaceful havens and bountiful harvests.

The concepts and practices described are relevant to all who seek to enjoy the opportunities and benefits of living in a Mediterranean climate to the full, whether their garden is around a villa or town house, a finca or country house, or restricted to the terraces of an apartment or village house.

The presentation of the concepts and practices are not prescriptive in terms of you should do this or that. Rather it is more in the form of a case history leaving the reader to identify what is relevant to their own situation in terms of the design and planting of their garden, their lifestyle and their attitude to natural or manufactured health. Look for new ideas from page one onwards.

We hope that you find the book a useful and stimulating read. If it stimulates you to consider making changes to the layout and plantings in your garden then our earlier books will help you do so. But naturally, where appropriate take advice from your medical practitioners.

Dick Handscombe August 2011

1. WHAT IS MEANT BY WELL?

Today it is generally recognised that there are four important dimensions and benefits of personal and family wellness – spiritual wellbeing, healthy bodies, healthy gastronomy, and improved economic wealth. Each and all can be achieved by developing this holistic view of personal and family wellness and aiming to achieve it through ones' own gardening and growing efforts.

- **Spiritual or mental well being** by developing a garden around a house or on an apartment terrace that is inspiring and relaxing, a place for quiet meditation or reading, a place to siesta as well as exercise, a place for enjoyable family eating as well as entertaining, a place to potter and be excited by plants, and overall enables escapism from the rat race of the 21st century.

- **Sustained good physical health** through the mental and physical effort exerted in designing, developing and maintaining the garden and the consumption of self grown ecological and chemical free fruit, flowers, herbs, vegetables, meats and eggs. Especially those with high levels of essential vitamins and minerals.

- **Gastronomic satisfaction** by growing a diversity of seasonal produce. Produce that when harvested and consumed at their best provide a continuously changing pallet of tastes, looks, colours, smells, textures and colour combinations that give constant satisfaction and motivation, and are uplifting physically and mentally. It is not difficult when home cooking from own produce to create meals now rarely found in local restaurants and in glamorous starred restaurants at an affordable price on a daily basis.

- **Economic well being** by producing an increasing percentage of your own flowering plants, foods and beverages in a creative garden environment. This reduces the cost of eating fresh ecological produce on each day of the year. Reducing not only the price but also the time and travelling costs of searching out fresh ecological produce. A great garden can also reduce the desire to constantly get into the car to go elsewhere for shopping entertainment or escapism, or to live on medications and vitamin/mineral supplements.

Each of these dimensions of living well, even very well, is expanded on in depth as you proceed through the sections of the book.

I became particularly interested in this holistic view of wellness following two cancer operations back in 1993 to remove a tumour in a salivary gland. The surgeon advised me that the form of cancer was slow growing and resistant to chemo and radiotherapy treatment should any cells have been left in the body to re-grow. Further he forecast that if cancer was to rear its head again it was likely to be in the lungs.

He suggested that it would therefore be a reasonable risk to have no treatments but rather retire early to my then holiday home in Spain to do two things. Live an active outdoor less stressful life working in the garden and walking the local mountains, and consume a Mediterranean Style diet using ecologically produced produce. I am forever grateful for his advice and have enjoyed gardening and living well in Spain ever since. But could not obtain Spanish private health insurance.

Before proceeding I would like to suggest that achieving good heath is something worth striving for, for yourself and your family. It can become a family's greatest wealth but it cannot be bought. It can only be achieved by day to day efforts. In the case of partnerships this requires a mutual recognition of each partners holistic wellness needs, and joint effort to achieve them. Fortunately there is so much in a garden and gardening that can prevent and cure.

2. A WELLNESS GARDEN ENVIRONMENT

From what has just been said the design and development of a holistic garden needs to take into account the current and likely future lifestyle, health, exercise, relaxation, eating, hobby and economic needs of the owners. With a combination of common sense, creativity and sensitivity during its design and development a great garden can be achieved, within a number of years, on both large and small areas. Including large rural plots, smaller urbanization plots, apartment and village house terraces, apartment terraces, inner patios and courtyards.

A potted garden history

In my case the development of the garden evolved as follows.

1987 to 1993

House purchased in a quiet rural valley for switch off breaks, away from a hectic international working life. Residence increased from 8 to 18 weeks a year. Emphasis on transforming four abandoned agricultural terraces into a manageable state. The focus was on developing four unique mini gardens with their own mission, style and plantings. The considerable physical work involved building dry stone Intermediate terraces and side raised beds, a network of stable paths and terraces overcoming the muddy tendencies of Spanish red clay to become a quagmire after rain and then become within days as hard as rock, repairing a 25 metre long metre high dry stone wall to use as the base for a rockery, and improving the soil in areas where we planned to have plants and trees. Hedges were planted on two sides that were not walled. Started to plant half the area with mountain herbs and traditional local plants. A token area of three square metres was set aside for vegetables from day one. Half the plot, a large flat terrace, was left for the first three years for the wild spring flowers to grow. Garden seen as my fitness camp with many tons of rocks wheel barrowed onto the site from where roads would be eventually built. Unexpectedly, retired early at end of year after the two cancer operations.

1994 to 1996

Moved alone to live in Spain full time. Garden the means of recuperating spiritually, mentally and physically not knowing whether had short or long life ahead.

Development and refinement of garden aimed at achieving the needs outlined shortly. Generally the completion of rock work and more intensive plantings.

As first pests appeared implemented ecological solutions.

1996 to 2005

Met up with future wife Clodagh. As she was looking after more than a dozen gardens I helped out as way to meet up especially during winter cutback time. Variety of plantings expanded as we had a few frost free years and ample cuttings from these other gardens. Experimented with subtropical plants for our own benefit and to support our evolving gardening writings. Seats set up in various tranquil corners to enjoy a rest or read while enjoying internal and external vistas.

Enjoyed wonderful large mangoes and even a pineapple.

Took on extra land to expand the growing of ecological vegetables and fruit. Cold frames and greenhouse set up to grow flowering plants and vegetables from seeds and cuttings.

After a study tour/walking holiday in Cuba started to keep chickens and rabbits for ecological meat and manures.

2005 to 2013

After the record breaking frosts of February 2005 we did not replace most of the plants we lost and moved back to our original planting objectives. In case we had another cold winter we now set up each November a temporary plastic green house to protect a succulent collection and more tender plants from a dining terrace close to the kitchen.

Took on an olive grove to rehabilitate, starting with a 90% pruning, to produce our own extra virgin cold pressed olive oil. In 2011 moved some vegetables back into garden.

The needs and objectives of the garden

Over the past twenty five years we have aimed to achieve the following in our holistic garden.

1. A garden that draws one into it, and like a magnet away from the house. Not something to be just viewed through a window or doorway.

2. A natural and continuous link from a plant full front porch and back covered terrace, mini gardens themselves, to the garden and into the visible natural countryside beyond.

3. A holistic garden that includes the growing of beneficial herbs, vegetables, fruits, edible flowers, eggs and light meats for a year round generally wellness diet. Yes like everyone we occasionally transgressed away from our wellness diet. But occasionally was not allowed to become a chronic risk.

4. A control over the cost of buying and maintaining plants by focusing on a mix of native and imported plants that are reasonably drought and frost resistance, and can be propagated by taking cuttings and collecting seeds. Initially, when a holiday home, plants were mainly from the mountainside and to be urbanized terraces. In early days there were few garden centres and they had far less choice than nowadays.

5. Mulch, mulch and mulch with compost, rocks, stones, chippings, volcanic ash etc to minimize moisture losses by capillary evaporation.

6. A mix of evergreen and deciduous, plants with a stimulating mix of leaf and bark colours as well as flower colours, and ensuring a good number of edibles and natures medicines conveniently to hand. Also important was to have uplifting seasonal plants in terms of sight perfume and taste.

7. It was decided before we purchased the half finished house that there would be no pool, no lawn, nor a permanent irrigation system to minimize water costs. Plants would need to be deep rooted to survive six to eight week breaks away from the property except between June and September in the early absentee gardener years.

8. For the first few years we were almost an isolated house surrounded on two sides by pine woods, one side by abandoned terraces and on the fourth side by a long established house and garden, on the other side of an earth track. At this stage we kept boundary plants low in order to benefit from sunrises and sunsets and the amazing population of butterflies and birds. Then urbanization came with houses on all sides and 150 pine trees felled. Then we started to block out the offending houses, which by then prevented us enjoying each sunset, with thick high boundary hedges and trees and enhanced the garden by using the third dimension of height to the full with stimulating climbers climbing over gazebos up walls and up through the green foliage of trees. Plantings that not only added colour and shade but also privacy, reduction in noise and chemical pollution from the street and neighbouring gardens, and a day time haven and nesting sites for birds. It's now a green oasis in an expanding urbanisation.

9. An attractive place for local wildlife to migrate to and live and survive safely, adding natural interest from dawn to beyond dusk. We have a good population of frogs, lizards, geckoes and birds but not the rarities of the early years. Sadly urbanization and some five years of aerial spraying of citrus trees reduced our summer butterfly population from several hundred a day to just a handful of weekly passers by and hedgehogs no longer breed in the compost heap.

10. A garden that includes a mix and balance of areas and features that are restful, stimulating or/and enhance the enjoyment of the garden, and a generally outdoor lifestyle. Ponds, fountains and an aviary are now essential features.

11. The preservation and enhancement of natural features such as large rocks, native trees, dry stone terrace walls and distant mountain vistas.

12. A balance between full sun, semi shade and dappled shade for the seasonal benefit of visiting family, plants and pets.

13. Use of variations and changes in light, shadow, colour tones and hues to achieve scenic and spiritual effects.

14. Provision of interesting areas for summer and winter top ups of vitamin D away from prying eyes.

15. A chemical free zone by using natural practices including ecological fertilizers insecticides

and fungicides, and avoiding the use of herbicides. Each of our earlier gardening books explain how this can be achieved economically. See appendix 3.

16. Provision for ecologically friendly al fresco cooking. Once we discovered and purchased the paella pan, tagines from Morocco, a Mexican oven, and a parabolic solar cooker the kitchen is less used and for ten years we have not barbecued.

17. Overall something that has a spiritual dimension to get one away from short term and long term chronic stress We discovered that a quieter but satisfying live is still possible and worth while in the 21st century.

18. To see the garden as a lifetime project that combines useful physical exercise, using and developing ones creative skills in the initial design and annual enhancements, developing and using ones sense of space in three dimensions and most importantly colour mixing and risk management. Regarding the latter there are ample opportunities for creating holistic style gardens in Spain that are not only beautiful but also productive in all seasons taking particular advantage of the two springs, Spring and Autumn. But in doing so one needs to recognize and take account of the many risks associated with Mediterranean gardening as discussed fully in Chapter 1.2 of 'Your Garden in Spain, the first book in our series of five related gardening books (see the appendix 3 at the back of this book for full details). Those risks include very varying micro climates, amazing ranges of highest and lowest rainfalls and temperatures, the soils and variety of possible flowering and edible plants.

19. To work the garden in a safe manner, including:
- A gentle warming up in the sequence of early tasks.
- The use of ergonomic tools to reduce the effort required and chance of strains and sprains.
- The wearing of a breathable straw hat when working in the sun.
- During the hottest months to only work early and late in the garden.

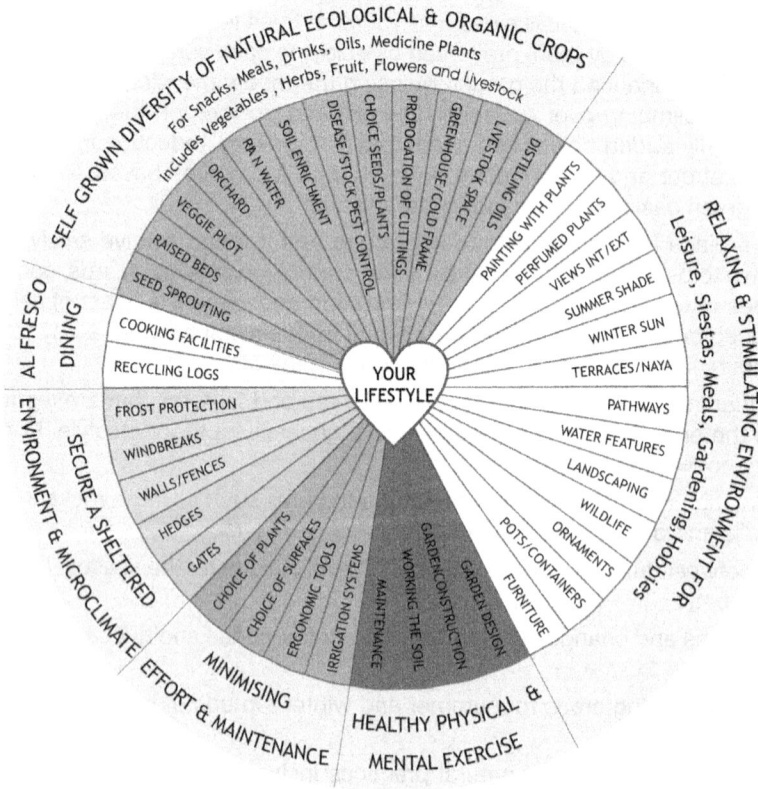

- To minimize the use of poisonous and spiky plants.
- Most importantly ban the use of inorganic chemical garden products.

20. Our framework for holistic gardening and living well presented on the previous page was first presented in our book *Growing Healthy Vegetables in Spain* is a summary of our original and evolved objectives, and final achievements.

3. SOME PERSONAL THOUGHTS ON EATING WELL

3.1 Only you can establish your own good health

From all that I have read listened to and observed about health for almost seventy five years, as a lay person with an analytical background, four fundamental things seem to make sense.

- Whether wanting to avoid or recover from poor health the most important factor is ones' own attitude to short and long term health.

- The lifestyle we are led to, or chose to follow, especially what we breath eat and drink, is a primary determinant of our personal health. Yet only you and I can decide what to eat, how it is prepared or purchased, fresh ingredients or processed foods, at what time of day and where, and whether on the run, socially with others or relaxed quietly alone in the garden.

- What we are taught about the relationship between health and good eating from the age of five to seventy five, in my case, is too often shallow confusing and obviously unconvincing in the Western world. Otherwise how come the world has so many overweight unfit persons. Many of whom are surviving on, prescribed and/or self purchased, corrective manufactured medications and harmful drugs while the long term successes of alternative natural based, often from birth to death, therapies of other civilisations are largely ignored and even banned by legislation. Will things change when Russia, China, India and Brazil overtake the dollar and euro based economies as a world power base? Changes have happened quickly in last half century but I expect I won't be around to know.

- With the rising costs of health care almost bankrupting nations why shouldn't it be every ones number one social responsibility to invest in their own wellness, before contributing time and money to other charities. Why shouldn't charity begin at home.

Together, sometimes in combination, today's main stream health service and yesterdays alternative health and medical advisers can hopefully put you on the right track or help you get back on track. But progress and success depends on your objectivity, determination and dedication to make it work. As we have read in WDDTY (What Doctors don't tell you) publications 'There are no free lunches to good health'.

Some time ago I discovered three notices on a range of bottles of vitamin supplements or top up pills.
- These are no substitute for a balanced diet.
- Don't exceed the recommended consumption.
- Discuss their use with your medical practitioner.

Yet they are sold by the billion and we have heard of persons who take up to two hundred plus food supplement pills a day not to cure current ailments but to strive for the 21st century doctor's dream – a waiting room full of 100 year old patients wanting to know what to take next! But as discussed in the next section *What do our bodies really require us to eat or drink?*

3.2 Dimensions of good and poor eating

Unfortunately our education, popular publications and television programmes rarely give us a simple memorable briefing on 'What we need to consume to grow and function well with good health from conception to the grave'. These days most emphasis of discussions about what we eat and drink seems to be about whether it makes us fatter or slimmer, the possible deficiencies of today's mass produced mono crop agricultural produce, the realities about processed and manufactured food stuffs, and the apparent benefits of food and medical supplements to make up for any deficiencies.

I prefer to go back to first principals because in earlier centuries many people lived healthily from what they grew or gathered/hunted in the surrounding countryside, and supplements as we know them today were unheard of. Personally I see good eating as meeting the following basic needs and poor eating as the cause of some basic problems that might result in the need for medical intervention if diets are not improved.

GOOD EATING requires that ones solid and liquid food intake is selected and balanced on a daily and weekly basis to provide for the following four fundamental needs.

1. The **Fuel** that provides the energy required for our brain, body functions and processes to operate effectively every second of the day and night and for us to go about our daily lives and exercise without exhaustion stress or damage.

2. The **Fertilizer** which, as with plants, enables our bodies to grow healthily when young and regenerate when growing older – this includes all body cells, muscles and bones, skin and hair etc.

3. The **Failure prevention mechanisms** that ensure that our mind, body parts and processes operate healthily at all times and that we become aware of deficiencies in time to take self help corrective actions.

4. The **Fun** of being able to really enjoy the intake of both basic and gastronomic snacks meals and drinks.

POOR EATING results in an excessive intake of an imbalance of poor quality and unhealthy foods and drinks which can cause the following.

1. The intake of **FUEL AND FILLER EXCESSES** which become stored as fat or excess retained water.

2. A **FERTILIZER EXCESS** that can result in faster than normal and undesirable expansive growth, obesity and in extreme cases stimulate and feed cancer and other unhealthy cells.

3. The stimulation of the **FAILURE AND BREAKDOWN** of the brain, mind, body parts and processes.

4. The **SHORT TERM BUT UNLASTING FUN** of an unhealthy, often gluttonous, lifestyle.

The choice between good and poor eating is not a privilege but one available to most of us in the developed world. For me, intending from 1993 to survive cancer by good eating rather than undertaking chemo and radio therapy treatments, the fundamental Mediterranean diet has been a good model to follow.

3.3 A holistic healthy Mediterranean diet

In 1993 when I was recommended to stop work and retire early to Spain to enjoy a Mediterranean diet it was difficult to determine what was the original healthy Mediterranean diet as various authors of articles on the subject took a narrow partisan view. The description of a framework for a Mediterranean diet was biased one way or another to promote particular products and services and failed to highlight that pre industrialisation an important factor was that the environment and what was eaten was chemical free.

Inevitably my own model is a personal interpretation of what I have read, heard and observed. It is as follows. I started with the premise that a description of the best of original Mediterranean diets needs to include all those things that a body would have taken in during a day week and month. The following seventeen elements were identified.

THE HOLISTIC MEDITERRANEAN DIET

- Fresh air – oxygen and aroma of nearby native herbs.
- Regular exercise – to collect and in many cases grow foods.
- Spring water – energised by natural vortexes and cascades.
- Fresh herbs - some for flavour, some recognised as being beneficial to health.
- Fresh vegetables – harvested each day whether grown or bought.
- Fresh fruits – harvested and eaten when at their best, often daily.
- Nuts – harvested from own trees or in the wild.
- Fresh fish – from the local sea, rivers or lakes.
- Some naturally reared meats – fresh, air dried or cured – the best and most eaten only on feast days.
- Artisan sheep and goat cheeses – own or locally produced.
- Sun dried vegetables, herbs, fruit, nuts and fish and meats – to eat raw or in prepared dishes out of season.
- Local red wine and grape juice – own, family or neighbours
- Local milk – goat or cow, own animals or local often milked at **the door.**
- Hillside honey – wild or hives – own or neighbours.
- Artisan breads – often from families local variety home grown grains – stone ground at local mill and whole meal.
- Olives and olive oil – often from own trees – own curing of olives and oil from local cold press.
- Natural colorants and flavourings – using natural features of the above ingredients -wide use of herbs, peppers, saffron for orange tints, and sun dried or mined salt.

That list made so much sense when first drawn up. I started by walking the herb scented mountains around our valley and filled the garden with aromatic plants.

Secondly I taste tested five local springs and collected drinking water from the two best ones.

Thirdly since most ingredients were once upon a time self grown, bartered or bought without travelling beyond the homestead, village or town I set out to do the same as discussed in Part Four.

The five exceptions cheese, fish, honey, wine, and cured ham I buy from like minded artisan producers except for fish which are mostly self caught on rod and line.

3.4 Some typical eating objectives

In spite of publications referring frequently to the traditional Mediterranean Diet everyone has their own objectives for eating and drinking.

Some consider the issue objectively and set firm objectives. Others by default, and without apparent reason, follow a fairly set programme of eating and drinking without necessarily recognising that they are doing so. In general the former group of people are aware of the need to live more healthily and the other group give little concern to the issue, believing that if things go wrong their medical adviser has something up their sleeves for every condition that might occur.

Typical objectives for the two groups of people might be as follows.

Objectives of the more healthy or health conscious.
1. To feel healthy.
2. Not to feel bloated.
3. To have energy throughout the day every day.
4. Have stamina for long walks/periods of exercise.
5. Maintain a comfortable weight.
6. Avoid manufactured chemicals in the form of:
a. Unnatural additives such as flavourings, aromas, tenderizers, fillers and preservatives.
b. Surface pollutants of fruit and vegetables from insecticides, fungicides, herbicides, foliar and root fertilizers.
c. Packing station fungicides, colourant washes and waxes.
d. Medicinal products.
e. Leaching from packaging materials.
7. Eat/drink preventively to avoid need for doctor visits.
8. Control alcohol intake and drink mainly water based drinks including fresh water and natural herbal infusions.
9. Avoid cravings for processed foods especially sweetened carbohydrates.
10. Not to get hunger pangs.
11. Eat what is most healthy for their blood group.
12. East well daily –at least as healthily and gastronomically as a good family restaurant that uses own, family or local eco produce.
13. Enjoyment of meals and snacks.
14. To generally sleep well even if eating late.
15. To not suffer indigestion.

Objectives of the less healthy or less health conscious.

1. Follow latest diet fad
2. Regular use of slimming pills
3. Eat fast food for speed and enjoyment
4. Drink tasty carbonated drinks
5. Rely on sleeping pills after heavy meals.
6. Rely on medicines and supplements to counteract deficiencies in diet.
7. Enjoy regular carbohydrate boosts to reduce hunger.
8. Mainly rely on processed foods.
9. Plan weekly/weekend binges and blowouts.
10. Starve mid week.
11. Ignore health advise.
12 Happy to be unfit and over weight.
13. Food is to fill. Not too worried about taste as this can be modified with salt and sauces.

We prefer to aim at the former through a Mediterranean style diet relying largely on home grown produce.

3.5 Typical side effects of poor eating

Daily one not only reads about the possible side effects of poor eating but can observe it from others around one and most importantly ones' own body. The following list is a start point.

- Weight gain or loss.
- Poor sleeping, lack of energy and hangovers.
- Lack of motivation and concentration.
- Dependence on drugs, vitamin and mineral substances and unhealthy soft or alcoholic drinks.
- Slow childhood development and growth.
- Development of unhealthy conditions.
- Slow recovery from unhealthy conditions and wounds.
- Rushed eating.
- Affects on children of the unhealthy.
- Dislike of good fruit and vegetables.
- Not keen to drink water or herbal infusions.

Before reading further where would you place yourself on the following scale?

I eat very unhealthily							I eat very healthily		
1	2	3	4	5	6	7	8	9	10

If you score to the left perhaps you could find room in your garden or on an apartment terrace to grow some more healthy foodstuffs on a regular basis, if necessary amongst the flowering plants cottage garden style.

3.6 Risks to availability of affordable healthy local food

Unfortunately unless you grow your own there are risks to the availability and cost of locally produced or even imported produce as illustrated below.

- Slowness of growers to switch back from chemical driven production to former but now improved ecological practices.
- Continued abandonment of small scale local agriculture on small plots around villages and towns as the low prices received by growers from commercial buyers do not cover their costs.
- Reclassification of agricultural land to industrial, urban and protected rural lands.
- Desertification as a result of felling trees, leaving land bare, overuse of chemicals, salination of wells and global warming.
- Middle East and Far East countries and China buying up the fertile land in Africa to grow produce for export to their own growing populations and Japan buying land in China.
- High transport and warehouse/chill room/frozen food store costs once produce is not sold direct to local customers and stores.
- The seeds of many traditional local varieties of vegetables, fruit and herbs are not being preserved for sale to commercial or home growers.
- The draconian EU control on the continued sale of some popular herbal treatments.
- Less stringent quality control in some exporting countries.
- More and more produce grown under plastic.
- Multi- handling reduces the natural freshness of produce. No chilling process can duplicate the impact of harvesting and immediately consuming a delicious fully ripe fruit.
- Much fruit is harvested before being fully ripe and may be treated to enable storage for several months before sale for consumption.

Our solution has been to grow more and more of our own produce as discussed in Part Four.

4. ACHIEVING SELF SUFFICIENCY IN WELLNESS FOODS

4.1 What do we need from what we eat and drink?

Most of us who garden on one scale or another realise that plants need carbon dioxide and oxygen from the air and soil based nutrients to grow from a seed to a mature healthy plant. These needs are summarised on the left hand side of the table opposite.

Healthy growth we regard as a combination of:

- Steady growth with the ability to avoid and withstand insect and fungicide attacks.
- Production of new healthy reproducible seeds.
- Production of internal nutrients that will be recycled to the earth through decaying leaves, and nitrogen fixation in the case of peas and beans, and in the case of edible plants their leaves, stems, fruits, seeds and roots become health creating foodstuffs for humans, domesticated animals and poultry, and wildlife.

If the nutrient intake becomes out of balance weak or stunted plants will result due to plants being grown in poor soil, given insufficient or too much water, achieving only low intakes from the air due to dirty leaves which clog the tiny pours through which they absorb nitrogen carbon dioxide and oxygen from the air and foliar feeds. If plants are fed with too much nitrogen they can grow too fast and become weak, especially if they are starved of phosphorus with aids the development of good root structures that search for moisture and nutrients in the soil. Growing this way they may have little resistance to pests and fungal diseases and soon need spraying with insecticides and fungicides to kill off the attackers. This can occur in industrial vegetable greenhouses or on vegetable plots when the gardener is more concerned with size than taste and texture. It also occurs in greenhouses where flowering plants are forced in order to speed up the preparation of ready for sale plants in full flower. In the worst cases the above ground structure of branches, leaves and flowering buds become too large for the root ball to maintain when first planted out in the garden. The result is that such plants need constant watching and care until they are established. Unfortunately this won't happen in all cases for the roots have been trained to live off constantly available nutrients in the irrigation water rather than needing to search for it in the open soil. That is why younger unforced plants whose roots are still growing and are not pot bound are a safer buy.

We humans and our pets and other domestic animals are no different.

As illustrated in the table opposite we also require regular balanced intakes of nutrients in the form of air, food and drink, from birth to the grave, if a long healthy life is to be achieved. If our hourly, daily and weekly intakes are out of balance then we can become exhausted even by moderate exercise, become overweight or anorexic and unnecessarily unhealthy. Luckily 'we are largely what we decide to eat and drink'. We have daily choices between Fast and Slow foods and drinks, between buying fruit and vegetables with residual chemicals on and in their skins or free of contaminants, meat forcibly raised with growth hormones and antibiotics or naturally fed home reared poultry and rabbits. Bottled and clean spring water is now preferred by most people in the industrialised world to recycled water contaminated with chemicals and medications that are not always taken out by water recycling/processing plants. These choices start at birth. Many babies react negatively to a substitution of dried milks for natural milks. Preferences for various types of food and drink develop through weaning and the style of eating allowed through infancy and puberty.

Unfortunately most of our educations have not emphasised what we need to be healthy and where we can best find the essential nutrients, vitamins and minerals for life time wellness. But we are so often told what is bad for us to eat, what the implications could be, and that the medical profession have an armoury of medications up their sleeves to help us when we get into trouble. So what can we do? Continue to eat unhealthily or change?

Our approach has been to grow our own healthy ecological foods and learn about their benefits to help us make choices about what to eat regularly. Unfortunately the information that we present in the following sections has taken some years to assemble and I suspect that many people give more attention to what the plants in the garden need to be healthy than to what they need in their own food and drink. We publish our current information now to aid others to understand more and possibly follow our path to self sufficiency. Today we really only need to purchase artisan eco produced cheeses cured hams and wines to live well in all respects.

The chart makes interesting reading! Our conclusion was that we should get to know more about which plants could act as a good source of nutrients and minerals for a healthy diet, and for priority growing. These are discussed in later sections.

Some essential needs for healthy plants and people

Substances	Required by plants for:	Required by people for:
Oxygen	To oxidize and extract energy from organic food molecules.	Breathing process and metabolism oxidation process
Carbon dioxide	Taken in at night and converted to organic molecules to build plant tissues and store energy	No, it is breathed out of body as a waste product
Water	Plant cell strength and rigidity and in soil to help roots extract substances	Body cell strength and rigidity and to maintain effective digestion process
Hydrogen	Aids photosynthesis, part of composition of carbon compounds	The most common element in body as part of water molecule
Calcium	Cell growth and rigidity, and resistance to diseases	Bone strength, teeth formation and maintenance, muscle and nerve operation, circulation of blood, release of hormones and enzymes
Carbon	Aids photosynthesis	Building block of fats, proteins, carbohydrates and DNA
Nitrogen	Development of plant structure – roots, stems, branches and leaves	Building block of muscles, gained from food not from breathing in
Phosphorus	Development of strong root structures	Development of skeletal structure, metabolism, DNA/RNA storage and transportation
Potassium	Development of flower buds, flowers, seed heads, fruit and drought and disease resistance	Control of acidity level, blood level, water balance, muscle contractions, cramps, nerve operation and protein metabolism
Sodium	Aids photosynthesis in some	Extra cellular fluid
Vitamin A	Seed germination of some plants	Eyesight, immunity to colds etc
Vitamins B types	As above	Effective working of enzymes in body
Vitamin C	As above	An important anti oxidant
Vitamin D types	As above	Aid absorption of calcium

Vitamin E	Protects chloroplasts from oxidation	Tocopherol, cell growth and health of bone marrow
Vitamin H	CO_2 transfer in photosynthesis	Biotin, metabolism and release of energy, cell health, reproduction
Vitamin M	Non identified in search	Folic acid, red blood cells
Vitamin P types	Pigments, nitrogen fixation	Bioflavanoids, brain, nerves
Vitamin K types	Energy transfer in photosynthesis	Control of blood clotting process
Magnesium	Chlorophyll formation and control to maintain green colour of plants	Growth/maintenance of bones, many body processes,blood pressure control, endurance levels, antioxidant
Sulphur	General plant and soil health, enhances extraction of minerals, on surface of leaves prevents fungal diseases	Efficient cellular use of oxygen, amino acid body building block
Iron	Prevents bleaching of leaves and helps chlorophyll creation	Hemoglobin formation and transportation of oxygen, good immune system and energy levels
Zinc	Prevents yellow on leaves	Enzyme activity and healthy immune system
Manganese	Prevents yellowing of leaves	Brain and enzyme activity, nerve health and joint lubrication
Selenium	Not essential, but need to include some to provide to humans	Antioxidant, cardiovascusaide health, controls diabetes side effects, arthritis, thyroid control
Boron	Aids development of cell structures and natural disease control	Healthy bones and joint function
Copper	Essential micro nutrient	Health red blood cells, nerve protection, connective tissues, cell energy
Molybdenum	Essential micro nutrient	Enzyme activity, alertness/concentration, liver health, male sexual function
Iodine	Stimulates growth of some plants	Function of thyroid gland, antioxidant and general health
Microbes	In soil/composts to convert substances into more easily extractable forms	In the gut to aid process of digestion and absorption of beneficial substances from foods
Fibre	To improve structure and water retention of soil	Aids digestion, healthy stomach and intestine, heart protection, insulin control

This table suggests that we should learn a little more about what is in the foods we consume to be happy that the diversity of what we eat achieves a balance between our various body needs and our enjoyment of food.

Hippocrates, a Greek philosopher, was obviously onto something when he said 'Let food be your medicine and your medicine your food'.

4.2 What have we done?

We have grown home produce for most of our lives. Encouraged by parents and grandparents we started when five years old, with mini gardens and school gardens and then expanded to containers and raised beds and eventually full sized vegetable and fruit gardens and allotments. However, we cut back on this when we first moved to Spain and grew just a few specialities for the valley in which we live was then fully self sufficient. Good vegetables meat edible flowers fruit and olive oil were always available for the resident families shops restaurants and visiting shoppers. The village had a reputation for quality produce at fair prices, to both the consumer and the grower, and some produce was still grown by traditional ecological methods.

However over twenty five years this self sufficiency with excess crops for sale outside the valley has largely disappeared, and most of what is still grown is no longer ecological but is totally dependent on chemical fertilizers, insecticides , fungicides and growth stimulators.

We therefore expanded the growing of our own produce to be able to be eat a healthy selection of vegetables, edible flowers, herbs, fruits eggs and meats on a daily basis throughout the year, and be sure that they had been grown ecologically. Today's diversity of produce helps us prepare gastronomic meals from tasty quality ingredients. Each harvested when at their best and ,very importantly these days with our declined pension and capital, at a significantly lower cost than purchasing such produce from local markets, shops or supermarkets. So we live healthily, gastronomically and economically without economising on the scale of meals we prepare for ourselves or when entertaining friends.

While expanding our own efforts we carried out in parallel experiments in the growing of crops in the kitchen, in the garage, in containers of various shapes and sizes and in raised beds in order to demonstrate to those who do not have sizeable gardens that much can still be grown in small spaces. These experiments led to chapters on the mini growing of vegetables and fruit included 'Growing Healthy Vegetables in Spain', 'Growing Healthy Fruit in Spain' and 'Apartment Gardening Mediterranean Style'.

So growing ones own produce is possible for all, including children and those unluckily enough to not have the energy and strength to cope with a full scale garden. In the sections that follow we summarise our current understanding of what is best to grow for the healthy eating and drinking of a Mediterranean style diet that can save money and hopefully result in less need for medical support.

When deciding what to grow and eat we did not follow prescribed diets aimed at calorie intake but rather concentrated on what could contribute to our short and long term health in terms of its vitamin, mineral, fibre and antioxidant content etc. The later especially important to me having had a cancer scare. We therefore started making notes of what we heard saw and read but inevitably it was not all summarised for easy access and memories fade as one ages. Summary sheets are therefore included in the following sections which describe what we have grown and harvested to eat. We started this as an aid to ourselves but thought it useful to share with others.

In general we eat a high in vitamins and minerals diet which is relatively low in carbohydrates but higher in proteins from beans and peas and our eco livestock.

Most days we avoid foods which Dr. Adamo in *Eat Right 4 Your Type* considers alien to my AB blood group and Clodagh's O group.

4.3 Healthy fruit and nuts we have grown or harvested for home consumption

It has become an international health fad that one should eat five to nine, varying by country, portions of fruit and vegetables a day. Seems to make sense, provided one has access to fruit and vegetables when at their best and ecologically grown. Unfortunately this is, like in many parts of Spain, just not possible unless one grows ones' own. Our book **Growing Healthy Fruits in Spain lists some 74 fruits from which to choose depending on your likes and dislikes and the microclimate of your garden.** In the table opposite we list fruits and nuts that we have grown or been able to harvest free elsewhere. Each has been grown ecologically. Some of their published claimed beneficial properties are indicated. We amazed ourselves by the diversity that we had been eating and the balance vitamins and minerals of that we had been inadvertently benefitting from. Those starred are the fifteen which we probably regard as our favourites from a combination of length of season, good to eat fresh, extent of our available harvest, extent of potential benefits, and can be dried or frozen for out of season use. The others we have enjoyed but they have smaller crops or were only possible when we had a series of hot frost less years. The most important thing is that we are able to eat several portions of fruit a day, mainly fresh. For many we have developed uses for many in salads, cold tapas, cooked dishes and drinks. Most are grown, or have been, within our garden. However the soft fruits are on our allotment and olives on a separate olive grove.

The first fruits we planted were a lemon, orange, mandarin and tangerine. Luckily our builder tipped us off to look out for a Lunar lemon tree, and accept no other. This variety is perpetual, having new flowers and ripe fruit though out the year. Of the other three citrus trees it has been the tangerine tree that has grown fastest and had the heaviest crops. This is fortune for tangerines are now being seen as a super fruit of the future.

When we first came to Spain we never expected to grow raspberries. However around 2000 we had a walking week in the Alpujarras and, surprise surprise, found them growing between 1400 and 2000 metres with plenty of irrigation water from melted snows, even in August. We negotiated two dozen plantlets from the family of a hotel we stayed in and took them back to the rather lower height of only 400 metres of our vegetable plot. Luckily we flood the plot with water from a channelled water distribution system. They took a couple of years to become established but from then onwards each year we have had sufficient new canes to extend our rows and pass on canes to friends. Amazingly we can normally harvest from mid May until December from the same plants. No one could tell us the variety.

Currently we are extending our rows of redcurrants and blackcurrants as it is easy to root cuttings here. The trick has been to enrich the soil before planting with rich compost and mulch with comfrey leaves which are high in potash.

Fruit trees have been grown around the garden and in containers. We have trialed a number of types in containers, especially when writing the Apartment Gardening Mediterranean Style book.

Fresh fruit juice from recently harvested fruits is especially delicious and nutritious.

We always had a couple of olive trees but more to protect the house from winter winds than maximization of crops. We always had sufficient to pickle in brine and herbs but not for oil. However a few years ago we realized the extent to which chemical insecticides, fungicides and herbicides were being used by local families and commercial growers so we took over and rehabilitated an abandoned olive grove in order to add home produced extra virgin cold pressed olive oil to our daily Mediterranean diet. Luckily a Spanish friend has an old style press with hessian mats.

No	Fruit	Apparent potential benefits we have become aware of over the years from readings and discussions.
1	Almonds *	Vit E B2, manganese, copper, phosphorus, healthy hair and teeth, respiration, brain, complexion, cholesterol
2	Apple	Help prevent cancer and Alzheimer's. For ladies aids bone density
3	Apricots	Vit C, Heart health, beta-carotene, calcium, potassium, silicon, iron, phosphorus
4	Avocado *	Vit E, anti oxidants, Helps with prostrate and breast cancers, eyes, heart, stroke prevention, cholesterol, anti oxidants, nutrient absorption
5	Azerolo	Vit C, liver, skin, cancer, immune system, fevers, headaches
6	Azofaifo /jajube	Vits A B C, cancer, sedative, anxiety/tension, muscle strength, liver, blood
7	Banana	Energy levels, depression, potassium prevents cramps, sight, bone strength

8	Blackberry*	Vits C E, antioxidants, eyes, heart, hemorrhoids, cancer, heart, mouth ulcers
9	Black currant	Vitamins, potassium, antioxidants
10	Cactus	Health giving flavonoids, wound recovery, reduction uric acid
11	Carob	Vitamin B's, c antioxidants, calcium, potassium, copper, manganese, fibre, energy boost, anti cramping, intestine and bowel functions. A very good rabbit food, also chew on walks!. Also hosts a tasty fungus.
12	Cherry*	Vit C, Prevents/soothes gout and arthritis, aids sleep and memory, slows aging, potassium, antioxidants
13	Elderberry	Vit A B C, beta carotene, vision, immune system, anti bacterial, heart health
14	Fig*	Potassium, memory, sex, hypertension, constipation, asthma, body renewal
15	Gooseberry	Vits A C, calcium, iron, phosphorus, bowel functions
16	Grape*	Vits A B C P PP K, phosphorus, iron, calcium,manganese,magnesium, enzymes
17	Grapefruit	Vits A B C D, folic acid, fibre, folic acid
18	Hickory/pecan nuts*	Vit E, antioxidants, mind/nervous system, heart, cholesterol
19	Joji berry*	Vit A, anti oxidants, anti aging, Alzheimer's
20	Kiwani/kiwi	Vit C E, fibre, potassium, copper, manganese, magnesium
21	Lemon*	Vits A B C P, vision, alkaline residues in body
22	Mango	Vits C E, anti cancerous beta carotene, potassium, copper, kidney stones, concentration, sex, digestion, cholesterol, sun burn protection
23	Mandarin	Vits A C, fibre, mouth cancer, protects cells and DNA from radiation
24	Medlar	Vit B C, anti oxidant, kidney stone, diarrhea, laxative
25	Mulberry	Vits A B C E K, minerals, blood vessels, potassium,iron, magnesium, Mn
26	Natal plum	Vits A B's C, protein, calcium, iron, manganese
27	Olives*	Vit E, iron, copper, fibre, energy, anti inflammatory,
28	Orange	Vit C, fibre, heart, blood pressure, pith anti cancerous
29	Papaya	Sap from leaves and stems removes skin lesions, beta carotene
30	Passion fruit	Muscle relaxation, anxiety reduction
31	Peach*	Vits A and C, beta-carotene, fibre, calcium, digestive and urinary systems
32	Pear	Vits A B C K, folic acid, calcium, potassium, copper, manganese
33	Persimmon	Vit A and C, Anti oxidant,fibre, sedative, minerals, skin blemishes, anti aging
34	Pineapple	Protein digestion, heart, sulphur
35	Plums	Anti oxidants, Vit C, fibre, eyes
36	Pomegranates*	Anti oxidants, anti cancerous and Alzheimer's,
37	Quince	Quince jelly to eat with cheese. Vit A, iron, fibre
38	Red currants	Vit C, iron, potassium, fibre
39	Raspberries*	Vit A and C, Antioxidant, vitamins, minerals – a Super Food
40	Rose hips	Vit C, vascular system
41	Strawberries cult/wild*	Vit C, anti oxidant, Vit C, blood sugar level
42	Strawberry tree	Antiseptic, diuretic, astringent
43	Tangerines*	Vit C and B's, fibres, potassium, folic acid, beta-carotene
44	Walnuts*	Vit E, fibre, calcium, magnesium, heart, blood circulation
45	Water melon*	Vit B C, beta carotene, pantothenic acid, magnesium, potassium, fibre, prostrate

4.4 Healthy vegetables we have grown

The table on page 19 has a selection of the hundred plus types of vegetables we have grown in Spain They have been selected on the basis of the following wellness benefits.

- We like eating them.
- Each has a significant content of beneficial vitamins and minerals.
- Combined in salads and cooked dishes they provide a phenomenal gold mine for our bodies.
- They provide a basis for seasonal diversity throughout the year.
- Few can be purchased really fresh or ecologically grown.
- Together with our herbs and fruit described in other sections we have no problem in meeting the recommended 5 to 9 portions a day of fruit and vegetables recommended by Spain and Australia respectively.
- They include plenty of antioxidants to combat aging and the possibility of cancer attacks, and include natural antibiotics together with the herbs.

How to grow the 36 listed and another seventy is described in our previous book *Growing Healthy Vegetables in Spain.*

The history of our growing of vegetables in Spain can be summarized as follows.

First six years when house used for eight to eighteen weeks a year.

Three one square metre raised beds were constructed on the west side of the house during the first summer to grow a few things that were not available in the village. Essentially Brussels sprouts for the Christmas visit but we only did so for two years as not really part of a Spanish diet, fine varieties of parsley, carrots, chives and red lettuce. Watered from rain water off the roof for many months. In the 1980's had a storm a month in summer.

Next five years after starting to live full time in Spain.

Although the agricultural lands were being increasingly abandoned it was still possible to buy good vegetables and villagers often gave presents. However there was a major changeover from the use of manures for fertilizer to chemicals and we, Clodagh by then living with me, became worried about the use of chemical fertilizers and excessive irrigation. Taste was being lost to size!.

In the summer of 1998 we decided to disappear for 50 days and walk from the Bay of Biscay to the Med through the wilderness and small villages of the Spanish Pyrenees. One thing we envied was villagers still producing old style ecological vegetables. On return home we set about trying to buy, rent or borrow a piece of land as an allotment. There were few plots suitable for starting to grow vegetables ecologically but within a couple of months an elderly Spanish friend negotiated a plot for us on the basis that we could use it free for life or until they wanted to build on it free. Sods law operated! Within four years it was built on but we first secured a new plot and moved the asparagus bed and raspberries over. As the plot was 800 square metres compared to the original 400 we had room to expand.

During this period the first edition of our book 'Your Garden in Spain included a section on growing vegetables, then but eighteen months later this was expanded into the separate book *Growing Healthy Vegetables in Spain.*

Next seven years until record breaking frosts of 2005

In expanding we grew more and more types and varieties and paid for seeds and water by selling vegetables to friends and a Michelin starred restaurant. The latter paying very well for early season mini ecological vegetables. A great idea but fame led to the restaurant moving away from our area to the centre of Valencia. We also expanded the soft fruit area.

Beyond 2005

The February frosts destroyed the collections of succulents and echiums we had around a series of four moderate sized ponds on four terraces linked by waterfalls on the East side of the house. We had intended to improve three of the ponds so we thought 'Is that the best use of the area as we age? '. The answer was no as we realized that one day we would not want the bother of using the allotment to grow more vegetables than we could eat ourselves. So the area was revamped into an area of deep raised beds which we started to use for local salad crops and special blocks of herbs such as nasturtiums, perilla, parsley mint and stevia. The latter as a natural alternative to sugar.

By 2010 thieving was starting in the open fields around our allotment and with the rapidly accelerating abandonment of the agricultural lands our allotment was no longer surrounded by other productive plots but by one and a half metre high weeds. The result was that the water channels we use to flood the allotment soon became full of weed seeds and natural weed control started to become a major problem. So we started to expend the soft fruit rows and plant Alfalfa for the rabbits instead of buying.

Then out of the blue we were contacted to write **Apartment Gardening Mediterranean Style.** As with the earlier books we did not want to write about things we had not done or seen done so we developed an upstairs three square metre terrace into a productive veggie plot with vegetables growing on a growing table , in a trough with trellis, in pots on the floor and in tiers of window boxes attached to a wall and the metal security door to the terrace. 21 vegetables were grown the first year. Even more productive than roof top gardens we had visited in Cuba in 2002. So we had good photos for the book but new gluts of veggies from our various trials and allotment.

2010 was the worst year for robberies, mainly on adjacent plots but we lost a whole crop of onions and more and more people knew about our collection of heritage tomatoes. So for 2011 they have been grown in a ten-tub veggie plot on a terrace in the garden along the lines of our description in *Growing Healthy Vegetables in Spain.*

2012 Onwards: I am seventy five in the Spring and Clodagh wishes to spend less time vegetable gardening. The plan is to therefore to now grow all our vegetables except for our productive row of asparagus and some squash around the house, The allotment will be used to expand our alfalfa production to feed the rabbits, maintain the comfrey beds to produce liquid fertilizers and feed to the chickens, and expand the soft fruit beds, fruit trees and grape vines.

Around the house I will maximize the productivity of the area of raised beds, the ten-tub vegetable plot started this year and the experimental three square metre terrace started two years ago. There will plenty to eat even though less varieties of tomatoes will be maintained.

Sprouting Seeds: One thing not mentioned is that we have always produced batches of sprouting seeds especially during winter months. We started in trays but now have an automatic sprouting machine that washes the sprouting seeds hourly. Over the years we have experimented with many varieties of seeds as explained fully in Section 2.3 of Growing Healthy Vegetables in Spain. These are especially beneficial from a vitamin point of view.

Some of the healthy vegetables we have grown in Spain

Those starred *would be our first choices if short of space.

No	Vegetable	Some of the apparent potential benefits we have become aware of over the years from readings and discussions
1*	Artichokes - globe	Vit C, iron, phosphorus, potassium,calcium, folic acid and fibre
2.*	Aubergines	Vits B1 B3 B5 B6, anthocyanins, manganese, copper, iron, potassium
3*	Beetroot	Manganese, betacyanin antioxidant, a liver cleanser
4*	Broccoli	Vits A C K, and folic acid
5*	Carrots	Vit A, and beta carotene
6*	Cut and come again leaves	Combined benefit of the Vitamins and minerals of a wide range of European and Asiatic leaf vegetables.
7*	Garlic	Vits C B5 B6, zinc, potassium, calcium, selenium, iron, copper, antioxidant
8*	Parsley	Vits A C K iron and folic acid

9*	Peas	Vits A C B1 K, potassium, phosphorous, manganese, copper, iron, zinc, fibre
10*	Onions	Vit A, sulphur and other anti oxidants
11*	Red lettuces	Vits C K, folic acid and antioxidants
12*	Swiss chard	Vits A C K and fibre
13*	Shitake mushrooms	Vits B C K, manganese, potassium and some protein, anti cancerous
14*	Tomatoes	Vit C, beta carotene antioxidant
15	Asparagus	Vits A B C K, zinc, manganese, selenium, arthritis, bones, digestion
16	Broad beans	Vits A C, potassium, protein, fibre, libido
17	Butternut squash	Vits A B, iron, zinc, copper, calcium, phosphorus, fibre, cholesterol, weight
18	Cauliflowers	Vits C B1 B3 B5 B6, manganese, copper, iron, immune system, prostrate
19*	Climbing/ low beans	Vits A B1 B6 , fibre, antioxidants, folates, iron, calcium, magnesium,
20	Courgettes	Vits A C B's, potassium, iron, manganese, phosphorus, zinc
21	Cucumbers	Vits A K, fibre, carotene antioxidants, potassium, blood pressure, brain
23	Fennel	Vit C B3, fibre, iron, potassium, magnesium, respiration, eyes, anemia,
24	Leeks	Vits A C E K, antioxidant, potassium, iron, calcium, manganese, folates
25	Jerusalem artichokes	Vit C, phosphorus, potassium, iron, metabolism, probiotic Intestinal health n.b Eating garlic reduces the potential flatulence problem
25	Mange tout peas	Vits A B C K, phosphorus, manganese, copper, iron, zinc, potassium, fibre
26	Melons - water	Vits A B's C, antioxidants, sodium, potassium, magnesium, hydrator
27	New potatoes	Vits A C B's, carotenes, iron, manganese, potassium, fibre, carbohydrates
28	Pea nuts	Vits B's E, calcium, iron, phosphorus, potassium, protein, body building
29	Peppers	Vit B's C, iron, potassium, manganese, magnesium, selenium, immune system
30	Purslane	Vits A B's C, Omega fatty acids, iron, magnesium, calcium, potassium
31	Radishes	Vits B C, fibre, folic acid, phosphorus, zinc, liver, stomach, kidney
32	Rocket	Vits A C K P, blood, stimulant, liver, sex
33	Romanesque	Vits C B's, manganese, copper, iron, bone strength, colds, lungs, brain
34	Sweet potato	Vits C B's, fibre, iron, phosphorus, magnesium, immunity booster,
35	Squash	Vits B1 C A, manganese
36	Sweet corn	Vits B1 B2 C, fibre, phosphorus, manganese, heart disease and cancer

4.5 GARLIC – The number one healthy vegetable or herb

Without doubt we regard garlic as the healthiest vegetable or herb that we grow and eat and therefore we eat it every day of the year in one form or another.

The reasons for the health benefits of this long domesticated herb are the rich mix of vitamins minerals and anti oxygenating agents found with the garlic bulb.
The main ones are:
Vitamins – C, B5 AND B6
Minerals - zinc, potassium, calcium, selenium, iron, copper
Anti oxidants – diethyl sulphides, allicin

The ways in which we use garlic are as follows.
1. Chopped finely in salads at breakfast lunch or dinner.
2. Pickled in brine with added herbs as a tapas and in salads.
3. Chopped/mashed with tomatoes for spreading on fresh or toasted bread to which a little olive oil has previously been spread. An alternative to this is to rub the surface of toasted bread with the cut face of a garlic clove and then do the same with half a tomato. This is very popular in Spain. In Greece stoned olives are mashed with the garlic and tomato. For convenience the olive oil can also be mixed in rather than coating the bread separately.
4. A thicker version of the above with less tomato creates a tasty tomato olive garlic pate for eating on slivers of toast for a tapas.
5. Hot and cold garlic based soups can be tasty and spicy for winter and summer days.
6. Garlic is one of the many ways of flavouring pickled olives. Cloves can be either mixed with the olives when placed in pickling brine or added to olive oil for marinating finished olives before eating. Herbs such as thyme and rosemary are normally added to the marinate.
7. One of our favourite ways of cooking trout is to open them up and debone them like a filleted kipper. The surface is then sprinkled with chopped garlic and parsley and coated with olive oil before cooking under the grill.
8. Likewise we normally sprinkle lamb chops with garlic and rosemary or thyme before grilling them. If cooking lamb shanks or a leg of lamb we brush the skin with olive oil and finely chopped garlic rosemary or thyme, or we slot half cloves into slits cut into the meat.
9. Added to casserole and tagine dishes for flavour
10. A touch is added to the minced meat used to make meat balls for paellas.
11. We tend not to make gravies or sauces but when we do a touch of garlic is a must.
12. We often have some crushed garlic in olive oil ready for adding to things cooked on the griddle and some crushed garlic in lemon juice to take first thing in the morning during the winter months to ward off colds and flu.
13. Tomato and onion jams are popular in various parts of Spain and we make some most years. We have also experimented with a garlic jam for cold mornings.
14. What one must not forget is that young garlic can be harvested to use the thin stalks chopped in salads as an alternative to chives, or at breakfast or lunch time as a filler for a winter omelette.
15. We have been advised that some Doctors still advocate the historic practice of eating a garlic clove a day, top or bottom. Since we use garlic daily we don't need to follow this practice.
16. However there is a special thing that we do every three years. That is to follow a garlic based body detox programme for several weeks. We were told about the detox programme by a goat herdsman/artisan cheese maker living in a cave house above the snow line on Gran Canaria. He had obtained it from a Tibetan Buddhist monastery in 1972. He recommended that we use it every five years but we do it every three years as we live a more hurly burly life than a Tibetan monk. The detox programme is described in appendix 1.

4.6 Healthy herbs we have grown and harvested

In the table on the next page we list most of the herbs we have grown and harvested every year or at times in our Spanish garden. Many are permanent features while some are grown annually from seed. Often seed saved from previous years. Some appeared previously in the section on vegetables for we use some in more than small amounts in salads and soups. For instance garlic fennel purslane and rocket. In the table we indicate how we have used them and indicate some of the benefits we believe we have gained or could gain if we had the need. More information can be found on the internet for all of the herbs listed if you are interested. For the purists I apologize for not including Latin botanical names but space was precious in producing an economic book on a self published basis. Perhaps if a publisher is interested in a fuller version this can be accommodated in the future. The important thing was to share some valuable practical ideas fast. In any case the common names are more widely known and almost all plants are recognized Mediterranean plants. Many of course were brought to Spain by conquering peoples moving from west to east over the millenniums since the bronze age and are widely recognized as Mediterranean plants. In most cases it is the common version of the plant that we use. But in others we have a permanent collection as with mints and basil. With basil we buy a collection every few years from the Chiltern seeds catalogue in order to have a variety of varied leaf shapes sizes colours and distinctly varied flavours. One year they offered over thirty varieties. This year we have less than normal, due to planned travels and time required for writing during the hottest months.

Herbs are grown in the following situations within the garden.

- Mixed into the general garden.

- Those from the local mountainsides on a twenty five metre long rockery.

- On dedicated raised beds such as a semi shaded three square metre raised bed dedicated to nasturtiums, a square metre bed dedicated to parsley and a half square metre bed dedicated to the mint collection. Each of the latter plants planted in a half buried plastic pot to control their spreading and mixing.

- In plastic pots in the dappled shade under a pergola covered with passion flowers. For instance Stone breaker (lepidium draba) and lemon balm.

- Along the side of the vegetable plot and raised beds. For instance chives.

- Kalenchoe (pinnata,daigremontiana,gastonis boniieri) In widow boxes on a railing on the way from the kitchen to the garden and hanging on the door from a bedroom to our three square metre experimental terrace veggie plot. I like nibbling them when grazing around the garden as they taste nice and are claimed to be anti cancerous. By the way these plants plus stevia, perilla, houttuynia for which we don't have a common name, willow herb (epilobium parviflorum) were sourced from the Spanish charity Dolca revolucio, Sweet Revolution. Plants can be obtained by mail order from www.dolcarevolucio.cat. I met the organizers at the Slow Food Terra Madre conference back in 2008 when attending as a guest on the basis of our vegetable and fruit books.

Naturally most herbs are used fresh but we do dry some leaves for winter and rainy day infusions use on our five tier Stockli drier. This is faster and safer than in the sun for many herbs when the overnight humidity is high or it's the rainy season.

We recognize that some of the above herbs can have side effects, for instance rue but the small number of leaves used in a three infusions a day for three days to recover from a sprained knee or ankle is minimal and we know of no faster cure.

As explained in the previous section the herb we use most of is garlic. It's a toss up whether it is a vegetable or a herb. And by the way the banana plant is officially a Himalayan mountain herb!

Code in table: S= Salads, dg= decorative garnishes, cd= cooked dishes, id= infusions/drinks, p= pot-pourrie.

No	Name	Indication of uses *					Indication of how we have used, or could use for own or garden health*
		s	dg	cd	id	p	
1	Anise	o	o	o	o	o	Digestion ,bad breath, coughs
2	Bay			o		o	Burn to get rid of smells
3	Basil	o	o	o	o		Uplifting, colds and flu, jet lag
4	Chives	o	o	o			Chewed raw internal parasites
5	Comfrey - russian						Not edible but: Poultice for gout, strains/sprains Also a great natural fertilizer in water*
6	Coriander	o		o			Calming, antioxidant, bone mass

#	Name	1	2	3	4	5	Uses
7	Cumin			o			Energy, immune system,iron
8	Dill	o	o	o			Antioxidant, preparing gravlak
10	Enchinacia				o		Colds, flu
11	Fennel	o	o	o	o	o	Anti inflammatory, a beetle attractor*
12	Garlic	o		o	o		Natural antibiotic, detoxes, insecticide
13	Garlic chives	o	o				Blood flow, healing wounds, antiseptic
14	Ginger	o		o	o		Colds and flu, nausea, cancer, painkiller
15	Good King Henry						Digestive system, metabolism, bowels,
16	Horse radish	o		o			Metabolism, tonsillitis, thyroid, aches
17	Hypericum				o		In olive oil for sprains/strains
18	Houttutunia				o		Roots for muscles, stomach ulcers
19	Marjoram	o	o	o		o	Calming nerves, insomnia, migraine
20	Kalanchoes	o	o		o		Anti cancerous, burn wounds, allergies
21	Lavender		o			o	Distil oil, body lotion,
22	Lemon balm	o	o		o	o	Stress, anxiety, sleep, indegestion
23	Lemon verbena	o	o	o	o	o	Refreshing summer drink, calming nerves
24	Mint -various	o	o	o	o	o	Digestive, hangover
25	Nasturtium	o	o				Antibiotic, general tonic, insecticidal properties*
26	Parsley	o	o	o	o		Kidney, chewed removes garlic odour
27	Perilla	o	o	o	o		Food poisoning, allergies, aging, panic
28	Purslane	o	o	o			Antioxidant, omega-3, skin condition
29	Rocket	o		o			Chewed cancels garlic odour
30	Rosemary	o	o	o	o	o	Memory, energy, rinse dark hair
31	Sorrel	o		o			Hypertension, anti aging
32	Stinging nettle			o	o		Spring tonic, hair rinse, urinary
33	Tarragon		o	o			Appetite stimulator, blood vessels
34	Rue				o		Strains and sprains
35	Sage –common		o	o	o	o	Antiseptic, infusion for hot flushes, gums
36	Sage -pineapple	o	o				Flowers stimulating colour and taste
37	Stevia*	o		o	o		Sweet substitute for sugar, diabetes
38	Thyme		o	o	o	o	Infusion for chest infections
39	Valerian				o		Insomnia, calming
40	Willow herb*	o			o		Sweet leaves, prostrate

N.B. Fresh grated horse radish with olive oil and a little lemon juice is extremely good with fish and meat dishes and raises ones metabolic rate. This is especially beneficial after a heavy meal.

It is so easy to grow in an unused corner that one wonders why more of us don't grow it. Read the label of contents on commercial bottles of horse radish sauce and you might do fast!

4.7 Growing and harvesting edible flowers

Many flowers have wellness uses as illustrated in the table below which lists edible flowers harvested from our garden or from hedgerows on walks. We gathered these ideas over the years as illustrated below. Naturally there are others but do check before you use something new that it is not poisonous.

- Helping father gather and crystallize violet flowers and rose petals for use on cakes.

- Helping grandmother harvest pumpkin flowers to stuff with for dinner.

- Noting what restaurants have garnished dishes with.

- Visiting a friend Joseph Palmies's horticultural business near Balaguer Cataluña which grows and distributes mini vegetables and edible flowers. The highlight was watching and chatting to a colourfully dressed greenhouse worker from Africa whose job was to wander with a wicker basket along the rows of flowering plants harvesting a diverse range of fresh flowers. We added a few to our list that day.

- Lunching on a plate of just colourful hibiscus flowers with just a light oil dressing when being entertained to lunch at the Botanic Garden outside Havana. We now add them to our summer salads and dry them for infusions.

- Experimenting with adding flowers to drinks and dishes. When we make up a four litre batch of Kombucha each of the seven bottles it produces is often flavoured with a different mix of dried flowers and dried fruit.

- I used to drink a lot of good coffee having once lived in Holland and having a neighbour who was a coffee importer in Spain. But Clodagh had had problems with drinking tea and coffee and for years had only drunk infusions of fresh or dried leaves or flowers. I therefore decided to do the same and soon felt better for it.

The first drink of the day is normally spring water from down the road, often with a slice of lemon, followed by an infusion of fresh mint or rosemary leaves, often with a few flowers attached. Mid afternoon in the summer is likely to be a jug of cooled lemon verbena flower and leaf infusion.

With such a variety of seasonal flowers in our Spanish garden we seem to pick flowers every day for one reason or another starting with jasmine flowers as we come through the gate. The jasmine plant which now climbs up through a tall bay tree was the first in the garden. Twenty five years ago the builder planted it alongside the entrance gate as a moving in present. He said that the scent of jasmine was a traditional welcome to residents and guests to Spanish homes and it also helped keep flies away and make a pleasant infusion.

Naturally since we consume small volumes of flowers compared to vegetables the benefits of the vitamins and minerals in flowers will be solely a top up.

However I think the following quote is very true.

'Flowers always make people better happier and more helpful for they are sunshine, food and medicine. Luther Burbank'.

Healthy edible flowers we have grown

The following table indicates the edible flowers that we have grown ecologically and or harvested for eating raw in salads (s), garnishing dishes (g), inclusion in cooked dishes (c), preparing hot or cold drinks (d) preparing drinks and home decoration as pot- pourris (p) to improve the air.

No	Name	Range of our uses					Potential benefits/notes
		s	g	c	d	p	
1	Anise	o	o	o	o	o	Use in homemade liquors
2	Artichoke - globe		o	o			Vit C, iron, phosphorus, potassium, calcium, fibre

#	Name						Notes
3	Begonia	o	o				Liver, toxin elimination
4	Borage	o	o		o	o	Add to Kombucha
5	Broccoli	o		o			Vits A C K and folic acid
6	Caper	o	o	o			Buds used as capers, fresh or pickled
7	Chives	o	o	o		o	See herbs section 4.6
8	Courgettes	o	o	o			(c) Stuff and steam, immune system, vision,
9	Cauliflower	O		O			See vegetables section 4.4
10	Coriander	O	O	O			Digestive, spicy
11	Dandelion	O	O				Add to kombucha and pasties
12	Day lily	O	O		O		Vit B, energy, hairs, nails
13	Dill	O	O	O			See herb section 4.6
14	Dianthus	O	O		O		Flavour drinks, used to make chartreuse
15	Elderflower	O	O		O		Add to Kombucha
16	Garlic	O	O	O			See vegetable sections 4.4/4.5
17	Hibiscus	O	O		O		Relaxant, cooling, blood pressure
18	Hollyhock	O	O	O			Colours, flavours and respiration
19	Lemon	O	O	O	O	O	Add to kombucha
20	Lavender	O	O		O	O	Calming, nerves
21	Marigold	O	O		O	O	Add to kombucha
22	Mint	O	O	O	O	O	Add to kombucha
23	Nasturtium	O	O				Peppery, eyes, anti cancer
24	Orange	O	O	O	O	O	Add to Kombucha
25	Oregano	O	O	O		O	Antiseptic, stimulant, general tonic, colds
26	Parsley	O	O	O			See herbs section 4.6
27	Passion flower		O	O	O		Add to kombucha
28	Rocket	O		O			See vegetable section 4.4
30	Romanesque			O			Manganese, copper, iron: Bones
31	Rosemary	O	O	O	O	O	See herb section 4.6
32	Rose	O	O	O	O	O	Make rose water for soothing eyes
33	Safron			O			Keep little we have for paellas
34	Sage	O	O	O	O	O	See herb section 4.6
35	Sage - pineapple	O	O			O	Add to Kombucha
36	Squash		O	O			Stuff and steam or bake, immune system
37	Sun Flower		O				Seeds as tapas, chicken feed
38	Thyme	O	O	O	O	O	See herb section 4.6
39	Violas	O	O		O	O	Hay fever, allergies, congestion, boils
40	Violet	O	O			O	Can candy, capillaries, varicose veins

4.8 Growing and harvesting healthy leaves

Half an hour ago, sitting under the branches of our Ginkgo Balboa tree revising some earlier sections, I suddenly remembered that this section focussed on wellness leaves from trees had not been written. So here we make up for that with this short but interesting section.

Tree for leaves	How used	Potential
Bay*	Infusion	Anti oxidant, lung cancer, insect repellent, flatulence, when burnt removes bad smells from room
Carob*	Leaves	Floated on top of brine above olives in bottles or barrel they prevent moulds from forming.
Ginkgo Balboa*	Infusion or chew	Memory and attention of the aging
Fig*	Infusion	Bronchitis, can help diabetics
Olive*	Infusion or mashed	Antioxidant, antibiotic, anti-aging, antioxidant, anti cancerous
Neem	Infusion	Insecticide, shampoo and mouth wash
Papaya	Sap from leaf stems	Skin blemishes including skin cancer
Pine*	Washed leaves	To make gravlax – pickled salmon or trout Anti oxidant, DNA protection
Hawthorn	Infusion	Reduce blood pressure
Eucalyptus	Inhale over bowl of leaves in hot water or wash wounds	Decongestant, cold, flu, antiseptic
Tila*	Infusion	A good night sleep – will use it tonight

The seven starred trees are permanent features in the garden.

A sapling neem tree was for a couple of years before felled by a frost. We knew it was a risk as we didn't have the right climate. On the Costa del Sol it might have lived longer.

We know that we are too cool in the spring to get a papaya tree fruiting the first year and they are felled by frost. Ten kilometres away on the coast it is possible. A friend has some very old fruit producing trees. However we try to have a tree in a pot each year for its tropical effect and the beneficial properties of the sap of the leaf stems. Having heard about this in Penang and Cuba I rubbed some on a twenty year old mole like lump on a cheek that at times had been bothersome. Within three days it was gone and a long thick ingrown hair had fallen out.

Hawthorn and eucalyptus tress grow just down the road. We use fresh evergreen leaves all the year round and dry deciduous leaves for winter use.

4.9 Healthy meats we have grown and harvested

Chickens hens make amazingly friendly and intelligent family pets. Indeed we started to keep three hens after seeing an adjacent passenger, on a Spanish express train, take a hen out of a basket to feed it between Cordoba and Barcelona.

It lived on her apartment terrace and generally produced an egg a day. Our immediate reaction was 'If she can we can!' So a run was built within a month in the shade under a spreading acacia tree planted to block out two houses being built.

The timing was great as the last supplier of organic eggs had just packed up. This made us think creatively. If eggs why not chickens to eat? Didn't take long to agree and another run was knocked up. Free range chickens were no longer available and those reared in the large multi storey chicken sheds, nick named chicken hotels, used to live for 90 days. Now at the same weights they go to the abattoirs in half that time having been fed on growth stimulators and antibiotics.

Just after we got back from a study tour and walking tour of Cuba we discovered four tame rabbits living in a nearby field looking a little sorry for themselves after a freezing night. We assumed that someone had lost them or a Christmas present had been let go. So we fetched a fish landing net and managed to catch them. Next day we visited the few occupied houses in the area and put notices up in attempt to find the owners. No joy so within a week they moved from a temporary home in the shed to two newly built hutches.

So now out of the blue we had the missing meats for making home grown Valencia Mountain paellas having grown 2.5 kilos of rice in an old bath the previous summer, and having all the herbs required in the garden and the vegetables on the allotment. Back in 2011 we wrote two articles describing all the herbs, vegetables, meats etc together with the history method of cooking etc. These have been expanded and published as Amazon Create Space and Kindle books.

The other things listed below grew from there. In total we eat an interesting range of tender ecological meats which have generally white flesh and are low in fats.

The list below indicates the wholesome meats that we have reared ecologically and eaten.

No	Name	Main benefits we have become aware of
1.	Chickens	Normally have two or three hens for eggs and fatten six hens or cockerels a year for eating. As grown on natural grains, including maize, plus green leaves give an exceptional taste to homemade Valencian Mountain paellas.
2	Partridges	Home grown game is deliciously tasty and tender. Fatten half a dozen a year for festive days. Eggs can also be used in cooked dishes.
3	Quail	Grow both small regular quail and the larger North African Blue quail that makes a fine meal. Eggs great for tapas and salads.
4	Turkey	Most years fatten one or two turkeys for Easter and Christmas. What a taste raised on spare greens and whole grains.
5	Rabbits	Aim to eat two rabbits a week. Range of recipes we have experimented with would make another book. For Dick's AB blood group said to be one the best meats for him to eat. Only the breeding rabbits have names. When young Dick lived well on his fathers' rabbits in wartime London.
6	Snails	Collect from countryside, olive grove, allotment and garden. Fed on rosemary herb leaves for three or four weeks before preparing to eat. Had an intention to construct a breeding unit but can't do everything. Said to be especially beneficial to aging men . High in protein and unsaturated fats. Prepared in a tasty herby sauce as in Northern Spain. Rather superior to snails with merely garlic butter and parsley English style!
7	Guinea Fowl	Occasionally fatten for a special meal.
8	Ducks	Occasionally raise a couple of duck.

All have been ecologically reared as illustrated below.

- All are fed on spare and past their best vegetables, plus whole and crushed grains.

- Onions and garlic waste act as natural antibiotics for the poultry.

- We now grow own eco alfalfa on part of the veggie plot to feed the rabbits. Have recently discovered that alfalfa leaves can be a tasty addition to our mixed salads.

- By the olive grove we have a carob tree. The very healthy beans are fed to young rabbits.

- The young leafy branches pruned from citrus and olive trees are a great treat for rabbits and healthy as we only use ecological sprays.

A by product from the meat production is manures for composting ready to recycle to the vegetable plot, orchard and olive grove.

What a change from twenty five years ago! From a self sufficient village and valley to a largely abandoned agricultural valley but with our self sufficient household that can eat well, even very well and gastronomically 365 days a year with not much effort.

It tied in with my motto, originally from the Davos Conference of 1978, 'Focus on the future I will be there for the rest of my life'. And it has already been much longer than expected in 1993.

4.10 Some other wellness things from the garden

Over the years we have picked up some other useful ideas that emanate from the garden that help us live well from the garden. This is a selection.

1. Cleaning kitchen tops – Wipe over with half a lemon.

2. Cleaning windows – Dilute vinegar is not only a useful ecological weed killer but vinegar and water is also a good way of cleaning windows and glass table tops.

3. Getting rid of smells – Burn a few dried bay leaves on a saucer. If you always cook with fresh leaves then dry a few and keep the handy in an airtight jar.

4. Avoiding mosquito problems – Plant lantana plants under windows to deter any from coming into the house., If there mosquitoes around the garden at home or on holiday and there are lantana plants in the garden rub leaves between your hands and then rub them over all bare skin. You can also put lantana leaves in a jar covered with olive oil to extract the active agents from the leaves and rub the solution on your skin when in danger. Also recognize that geckoes are very useful animals around the outside of the house as they hunt any flying insect to eat. Encourage them to live around a covered terrace where you sit in the evening with lights on by hanging bunches of herbs from the garden in the upper corners. Rosemary or lavender work well.

5. Getting rid of ants – If you have purchased a box or bag of yellow sulphur, not copper sulphate, powder to dust fruit vegetable plants, such as tomatoes grapes melons courgettes and squash, to control mildew and other fungi attacks the same powder can be dusted lightly over ant runs and entrances to nests. This will kill the ants ecologically and will cause no harm to pets. A kilo costs only around two euros.

6. If you use canes, perhaps cut from your own plants, that are of a height that could cause face or eye injuries cover the top ends with empty washed out small plastic garden product bottles or mini water bottles.

7. Dried sage leaves mixed with salt make a good tooth cleaner. Sage leaves alone rubbed on receding gums help keep them healthy.

8. If you burn yourself the fleshy centre of an aloe vera leaf will five instant pain relief and speed recovery.

9. Marigold flowers in olive oil produce a soothing morning oiol.

10. Distill lavender flowers to produce some lavender oil and several bottles of fresh lavender water. Clodagh uses it in the shower instead of shower gels that include chemicals. Clodagh mixes the lavender oil into olive oil as a natural skin lotion. When we walked across Spain via the Pyrennes for 52 days from the Bay of Biscay to the Med only a small bottle was carried for weight. When It emptied friendly chefs in village restaurants topped it up with olive oil with amusement and Clodagh added the drops of lavender oil.

11. Good quality compost by composting all vegetable waste that livestock can't eat and shredded cutback material from the flower garden.

12. Edible colourants from what you grow. For instance tomatoes, beetroot, Swiss shard, hibiscus flowers, saffron, cumin, blackberries, oranges, nasturtiums.

13. Tasty vitamin rich home made whole grain bread with added nuts and dried fruits and herbs.

14. Cut flowers for the dining table and lounge.

15. Cleaning copper - rub with half a lemon.

16. Cleaning chopping boards - rub over with half a lemon.

5. Holistic gastronomy

5.1 Gastronomy versus gluttony

In Section 1 **Gastronomic satisfaction** was introduced as one of the four pillars of personal and family wellness. But what does that mean in practice for too often gastronomy is these days confused with gluttony. The New Oxford Dictionary of English defines gastronomy as the art of choosing, cooking and eating good food and a gastronome as a gourmet, a person who has a discerning pallet. Therefore someone who searches out good fresh produce for home use and when eating out prefers somewhere where fresh produce, perhaps home grown by the restaurant, and local artisan traditional specialities are used in preparing both fresh and cooked dishes. To this we would add someone who gains gastronomic satisfaction from seeing and eating an individual dish, even an individual tapas in Spain, just as much as in a several course meal.

Unfortunately when one visits some restaurants the special offer is sometimes not a special dish or series of dishes prepared from fresh local produce but a multi course menu of dishes prepared in advance and heated up in a microwave and rarely from fresh ingredients still full of the taste, textures and natural nutrients, vitamins and minerals as harvested, or slaughtered if meat or fish.

Further if one views the average supermarket trolley it does contain fresh vegetables and fruit including fruit for juicing, the days catch of fish and recently locally butchered meat but rather is full of a multitude of factory produced processed foods many with a microwave sticker on the packet and drinks that include juices that were first concentrated and needed added vitamins and mineral in order to make so called health claims. Just the fodder for today's gourmands who enjoy eating for the sake of it and often eat too much. Becoming physically and perhaps mentally uncomfortable in the short term and obese if gormandizing is frequent, even daily. The New Oxford English Dictionary defines gourmandizising as good eating but also eating greedily.

Naturally good needs to be defined as good can mean a wide variety of things depending on ones eating habits. As highlighted throughout the book I regard good as inferring beneficial for ones health as well as satisfying ones gastronomic taste buds. Unfortunately the expression 'This is good!' too often infers that a foodstuff satisfies a desire for sweet and salty foods and an immediate filling of the stomach. So there are overlaps, important overlaps from a wellness point of view, between Gourmet and Gourmand and good and good.

Amazingly in a world obsessed by obesity which is starting to put family, national health service and even national finances at risk there appears to be little concerted action to reverse the trend. The Slow Food organisation makes progress in some countries and regions but not always substantially. A Slow Food status can be granted to restaurants that source their fresh ingredients from growers and catchers within a 100 kilometre catchment area of the restaurant. But too frequently within that catchment area, especially along the Mediterranean coast, village after village has been steadily abandoning local agriculture for two or three decades, both for the market and the home. The main beneficiary as been the industrialised growing of vegetables under plastic. But there are now signs that more and more families are starting again to grow at least some of their own vegetables and re-prune some surviving fruit trees. Interestingly the one thing that has been continued while much else is lost is keeping olive groves going for own consumption, often hunting out an ancient cold press to produce the olive oil. But as at the commercial level much oil now depends on chemicals and tree shakers.

Some schools are attempting to stimulate an interest among children in growing something themselves and better eating. But what of the parents? A couple of years ago I walked 150 kilometres in five days to celebrate my 74th birthday. At lunch time I enjoyed a bag of home produced dried fruit and energy biscuits containing no unnatural additions and chewed some rosemary leaves for the energy giving oil. One friend unpacked a line of plastic containers of chopped onions, salad leaves and local cheeses and chorizo. The other two dined largely on sugar and additive rich biscuits and donuts.

5.2 The dimensions of holistic gastronomy for wellness

Looking ahead we hope that this book stimulates more people to :

- Not only look out for fresh ecologically grown produce but grow at least some of your own. As said earlier apartment terraces as well as small plots in gardens can be amazingly productive and cost effective.

- To grow as a priority those foods that contain the most beneficial vitamins and minerals, the best tastes and textures, and look and smell appetising.

- Again enjoy seasonal variations in diet. There is so much joy in harvesting inexpensive fresh asparagus daily for two months than being able to purchase travel weary imported bunches on each day of the year.

- Where possible grow traditional Mediterranean heirloom and heritage varieties of fruit, herbs, vegetables, edible flowers, chickens and rabbits as well as generally planting traditional Mediterranean flowering plants and trees.

- To focus on diversity of fresh ingredients and less on calculating calorie values. In reality the importance is to be energetic, look good for your age, free from unnatural medications and healthy aids and a sensible weight for your build.

- To harvest produce when at its best and fresh.

- To convert what you grow into fresh and cooked dishes in a manner that minimises the loss of the original nutrients, vitamins and minerals.

- To use healthy cooking methods, especially those that enable al fresco cooking. We minimise the boiling and frying of produce and for ten years have not had a barbecue in the garden. Our cooking apparatuses are as follows.

Our methods for preparing wholesome dishes

1. Raw torn and cut up mixtures for salads.

2. Parabolic solar cooker using heavy casseroles and a small paella pan.

3. Mexican oven for slow cooking of lamb shanks and baked potatoes.

4. Heavy casseroles for slow simmering on electric hob.

5. Three tier steamer on electric hob for vegetables, rabbit and fish.

6. Wok for stir fried or steamed vegetable mixes or meat and fish curries.

7. Two earthen ware tagines which cook slowly over clay pots of charcoal.

8. Heavy omelet pan on hob.

9. Paella pan for rice dishes and poached trout.

10. Five tier tray dryer with timer and air temperature controls to dry herbs, vegetables, fruit and dried snacks.

11. A home built wood fired oven – but with the above we rarely use!

- To use the natural colours and flavours of your home grown produce rather than artificial additives. Become more aware of the extent of additives in purchased processed products. They can include fillers, sweeteners, flavourings, colourants, residual growth hormones, surface waxes, fungicides, preservatives and water. I remember from the years I spent in the food industry the then importance of water content and fillers on profitability. It is unlikely that this has changed.

- Lastly do enjoy your wellness breakfast, snacks, lunch, dinner, tapas, dinner and sundowners etc within your green but colourful holistic garden with its fresh air, perfume, peace, but with relaxing and stimulating water and wildlife noises, great internal and external vistas, shade and sunny areas and of cause productive growing areas. I enjoy wandering round the garden grazing for snacks. A leaf of this and that beneficial herb, checking the ripeness of seasonal fruit and vegetables, and collecting the days eggs.

5.3 Where do you stand today?

If Spain is slow off the mark what about other Mediterranean countries. Italy, the birth place of the Slow Food organisation, is making considerable progress in making people aware of the opportunity of becoming close to producers, often stimulated by the book Slow Food Nation'. In this book the president of Slow Food, Carlo Petrini dreams, rather looks forward to, a new generation of wiser Gastronomes concerned with not only protecting and using the otherwise dying artisan products around the world but with also using locally produced produce and products in the home , schools, restaurants, hotels and hospitals etc, and by laying down personal standards and buying habits. Unfortunately the book nor the Terra Madre international conference and Turin Food Fair that I took part in back in 2008 emphasised sufficiently the natural wellness benefits of what one can grow and eat, even if only having small spaces available.

The need to do so was the main driving force of this book *Living Well from Our Mediterranean Garden*. The self audit that follows has been devised to help you evaluate the state of your personal thoughts and actions. The first draft was in my pocket at Terra Madre 2008 to evaluate the concept, but other priorities have prevented it's publication until now. Work through it factor by factor. Then add up your points and see how you match the four types of Gastronomes described. This is a first working draft of the audit. It can obviously be improved so your thoughts for improving it will be welcome via gastronome2@hotmail.com.

Factor	Tick which of the four statements alongside each factor best describes your recent/current action. If need be score half points			
	Score : 0	Score: 1	Score: 2	Score: 4
1.View of gastronomic eating?	Unadulterated gluttony from a dish or multi course meal that bloats, overfills, intoxicates and likely to put on weight	A special meal for a special occasion , rich ingredients and high calories for kicks as not a daily occurrence.	Satisfying balanced meal capable of being eaten without feeling under the weather. No heart burn, bloating or hangover.	Very satisfying deliciously tasting dish or meal that makes one feel special without unwanted side effects.
2. How often do you eat according to column four above?	Never	Rarely	Frequently	Daily
3. Extent of eating healthily from own produce from garden, apartment terrace or allotment?	Produce and eat no own produce	Use the occasional sprig of herbs and bay leaves	Harvest several times a week	Daily harvests of diverse mix of edible herbs, flowers, vegetables and fruit
4. Source of meat and fish if eaten?	Anywhere as long as it's inexpensive. Nothing home grown.	Selective purchase from supermarket without knowing source.	Purchase from local eco producer or local fishery. Have eco fed hens for own eggs.	Own eco reared produce or local eco farmer. Fish generally self caught from unpolluted waters.
5. Concern about source of ingredients in your meals?	Think worrying about E additives and sources is a lot of rubbish.	Buy mainly processed mass produced foods but look for eco foods for occasional treats.	Home produce half of what we eat, balance from local growers and farmers markets. Avoid products with E additives.	Aim to use mainly produce grown and raised in own garden or small holding with balance from local artisan eco sources.
6. Where do ingredients normally come from?	Don't really know but if see imported non seasonal things will often buy.	Very little is genuinely local produce. Much from other regions and imported.	Some own garden/ apartment terrace and rest mainly from local villagers. Rarely purchase imported out of season produce.	Over 80% own garden/ allotment or grown and raised in village or barrio of town. Concerned about quality and food miles.

7. Normally how fresh are your fruit and vegetable ingredients?	Don't know and not concerned. Generally use packed processed, tinned, bottled and frozen foods. Eat in cheapest fast food outlets.	Generally purchase pre-packed fruit and vegetables and watch out for end of shelf life bargains.	Becoming concerned about freshness of foodstuffs and are searching out market .local growers and growing a few things ourselves.	Harvest own daily, often within an hour or less of eating. When eating out try to search out establishments that grow own or source locally from growers direct or in local market.
8. Concern about healthiness of ingredients in daily diet?	Would not take an interest unless a medical practitioner demanded that I change my diet and lifestyle because of a dangerous health condition.	Becoming conscious of the risk I am taking with my diet.	Becoming concerned and now reading labels on processed food labels and not purchasing potentially risky items.	Ensure that each meal includes mainly foods with high beneficial vitamin, mineral anti-oxidant and low fat content.
9. Protection of bio diversity?	Grow and rear nothing.	Grow a few things but little concern for what the breeds are.	Starting to trace traditional vegetable and fruit varieties to plant up and grow.	Attempt to grow most things from traditional heirloom and heritage varieties and breeds.
10. How do you prefer your food to be cooked?	Accept whatever is served – not really concerned. If cooking for self normally use a deep fat fryer and microwave oven.	Generally fast cooking. Have rushed life and eating well not really important except at weekends when take pleasure in cooking better.	Eating more salads and starting to question how food has been produced when eating out and in meal preparation at home.	Raw or slowly cooked depending on recipe and ingredients.
11. How do you like your meals to be sequenced	Grasp what is available on the run when have time. Accept inevitable indigestion.	Skip breakfast binge. Take a working lunch and toasted sandwich dinner while watching favourite scheduled TV programme.	Starting to better organise timing and sequencing of foodstuffs within a menu.	Enjoy three good meals a day at regular times. Maximise pleasure by ensuring that the various dishes and drinks are eaten/drunk in the sequence in which the body can best digest and process without unpleasant side effects.

12. Recycling of waste?	All goes into general waste bin.	Have started a compost heap or mini waste digester and put some kitchen waste into it if I remember. Rest goes into general waste bin.	Most green waste goes into compost heap or digester. Rest into general food waste bin with other kitchen waste.	Healthy items fed to poultry and rabbits, other green waste goes into compost heap and only waste meat and fish into dedicated food waste bin.

Now go back to the beginning of the self audit and add up your scores. Then compare your total score with the table below.

What was your score?	Observations	Verdict!
33 - 48	Obviously you enjoy only good quality food, produced at home or locally by artisan and ecological means.	A new style GASTRONOME with focus on total wellness
17 - 32	Still enjoy a blow out but beginning to realise how much one eats is poor in quality but satisfies with volume.	An old style GASTRONOME with focus on quality and quantity
0 - 16	Clearly a fast food addict with little concern about what is happening in the food supply industry.	A FAST FOOD ADDICT

6. WHAT HAVE BEEN OUR BENEFITS?

What have been my and Clodaghs' benefits from developing an holistic approach to gardening and living well from our own ecological harvests and cooking? That's an interesting question. Need to think about that as it has become normal to day by day do the things we have described. Well we have brain dumped the following.

1. Health, fitness and energy.
2. A very diverse exciting and healthy diet.
3. Probably vegetables with more nutrients than many produced or purchased commercially.
4. Less stress about what we eat and drink.
5. Less time cooking.
6. Achievement of our ongoing aim to eat as well at home as in a traditional family restaurant that uses family grown ecological produce – unfortunately difficult to find these days.
7. Less expensive basic and luxury foods and drinks.
8. Less money spent on travelling to and in some cases having to pay to park to buy food at markets, local shops and supermarkets.
9. Less waste from having to buy more than you can use while still shop fresh.
10. Lest waste from not being able to eat 'shop fresh' but not yet ripe fresh fruit that often does not ripen properly after purchase.
11. Not having to eat out to eat well.
12. Less spent on expensive snacks eaten at home or when out.
13. No need to purchase vitamin and or mineral supplements.
14. No need to buy over the counter or prescribed medications.

15. No need to visit traditional, main stream or new high technology alternative medical practitioners.
16. Very rarely side effects from what we mix and match from the total ingredients available to us.
17. No time queuing up at the local Medical Centre.
18. Not consuming unnatural food fillers, colorants, flavourings, textures, surface waxes, preservatives.
19. No need to cut back on the extent or quality of our food in retirement, even with a reducing income.
20. Much less shopping time etc provides time to sow, plant and grow the wellness garden.
21. We hope an anti aging diet without having to resort to a plate of medicinal and health supplement capsules on a side plate as the first *tapas* of a meal.

Which of these benefits would you like to achieve?

7.0 THE WAY AHEAD. WHAT SHOULD I DO?

I have read through the book 'Living well from our Mediterranean Garden' and feel that I should start to do something fast to get me going. But where do I start and what could I include in a more comprehensive longer term programme?

It makes sense that you start by writing down what you now consider to be the good and bad things about how you currently eat and drink and what you currently grow and/or produce yourself.

The good things about how I eat and drink	The bad things about how I eat and drink
1.	1.
2.	2.
3.	3.
4.	4.
5.	5.
6.	6.
7.	7.
8.	8.
9.	9.
10.	10.

The good things about what I/we grow today	The bad things about what I/we grow today
1.	1.
2.	2.
3.	3.
4.	4.
5.	5.
6.	6.
7.	7.
8.	8.
9.	9.
10.	10.

The next thing is to list the things that you could do to sustain reinforce and extend the 'good things' that you already do well, and then things that you could do to overcome the 'bad things' about what you currently consume and the extent of your current self sufficiency.

Then consider the relative benefits of taking each possible action on your overall 'wellness' of living.

Things I would like to try and do	Potential benefit to my health H, M, L	Potential benefit to my enjoyment of eating H, M, L	Ease of taking the action H, M, L	Affordability of taking the action H, M, L	Overall priority for each action H, M, L
1.					
2.					
3.					
4.					
5.					
6.					
7.					
8.					
9.					
10.					

Code: H=High, M=Medium, L=Low

There may be more than ten things you would like to do but initially concentrate on a few things that score four highs to ensure that you get things moving in an immediately beneficial cost effective manner.

Maybe you feel you need to involve others in the changes to work with you to maintain your motivations, to give a helping hand with the work involved, to monitor progress, to share the successes and failure and quietly console each other over any lapses. Naturally spouses, family and friends could be involved.

Within the family the more members you involve the more chance of synergy between everyone's likes and dislikes. Children may at last understand what vegetables and fruit should really taste like and volunteer to help grow them as we started many decades ago.

The concept of Growing Circles may be helpful in the neighbourhood. See article in November 2009 archives of www.gardenspain.com for details. Circle members could be:

a. A family group or group of neighbours or friends living in:
   • The same block of flats – especially on the same or adjacent floors.
   • The same urbanisation – especially if in the same street or zone.
   • The same village – especially if in the same street or area.

b. Small groups from a school or local gardening club. In each case individual members or pairs of members would grow just one or two crops on behalf of all members which would be exchanged for produce grown by others.

We would love to hear of some of your successes in a year's time. Just drop us a line via www.gardeninginspain.com. In the meantime our earlier gardening books are available to give you detailed guidance and support.

• Your Garden in Spain ISBN 978-84-89954-670
• Apartment Gardening Mediterranean Style ISBN 978-84-89954-86-1
• Growing Healthy Fruit in Spain ISBN 978-84-89954-62-5
• Growing Healthy Vegetables in Spain ISBN 978-84-89954-53-3

Just remember that if you are under medical supervision and/or medication it is wise to discuss your plans for diet changes with your medical adviser.

Happy holistic gardening for wellness!

Appendix 1. The Tibetan detox programme

1. Mix 350 grams per person of finely chopped garlic with a quarter of a litre of a good quality aguardiente in a glass jar. Seal and shake well before placing in the fridge for ten days.

2. Strain the liquid after these ten days and then place in the fridge for a further two days. Then strain the liquid through a fine sieve and crush the garlic mash to squeeze out as much residual liquid as possible.

3. You are then ready to commence the detox programme.

4. For the next ten days transfer the following number of drops of the garlic extract with a dropper into a little water and drink before breakfast lunch and dinner.

Day	Breakfast	Lunch	Dinner
1	1	2	3
2	4	5	6
3	7	8	9
4	10	11	12
5	13	14	15
6	16	17	18
7	12	11	10
8	9	8	7
9	6	5	4
10	3	2	1
11	15	25	25
12	25	25	25
13	25	25	25

Then continue with 25 drops before each meal until all the liquid has been used.

The benefits claimed for the above programme on the document given to us by the goat herdsman are a cleaning of dissolved fats from the body and reduction of deposited fats, improved metabolism, greater elasticity of blood vessels, some weight loss towards normal weight, thinning of coagulated blood, healing of diaphragm, reduction of heart related deceases such as arteriosclerosis, isquemia, hypertension, sinusitis, throat and lung illnesses, disappearance of headaches, thrombosis, arthritis and rheumatism. Also said to be a cure for gastritis, stomach ulcers and haemorrhoids, reduction of internal and external cancers, plus problems of hearing and sight. In essence a curing programme and recuperation for the entire organism of the body.

Whether all can be proven or not it was sufficient to persuade us, that one way or another, there would benefits if we followed the programme.

Naturally with the above programme it's worth growing some ecological garlic each year.

Luckily young 'tierna' garlic can be easily grown in pots or window boxes for apartment dwellers.

It is interesting that until the 17th century the UK garlic was apparently as popular in England as the rest of Europe for its health properties. However the Hanoverian Kings banned it from the court, to appear cleaner than the French court, and garlic became a *don't use* vegetable down through the middle and lower strata of society.

Appendix 2. Some books we have found interesting

Over the years we have read the following books and retained them to refer to from time to time when our memories lapse or we need to explore something we have not thought of doing before or know little or nothing about.

1. Eat right 4 your type, Dr Peter Adamo and Catherine Whitney,1966, ISBN 039914255 X
2. Food for thought, Vernon Coleman, European Medical Journal, 2000, ISBN 1898947 97K
3. The Field, Lynne McTaggart, Harper Collins, 2001, ISBN 0722537646
4. Calendario Lunar, Michael Gross, Annual editions, Artus Porta Manresa, ISBN 97884936010
5. Aromatherapy for Women, Maggie Tisserand, Thorsons, 1985, ISBN 0892816287
6. How to live longer, Vernon Coleman, European Medical Journal, 2001, ISBN 18998947244
7. Nature Doctor, Alfred Vogel, Mainstream Publishing, 1989, ISBN 1851582746
8. Slow Food Nation, Carlo Petrini, Rizzoli, 2005, ISBN 9780847829453
9. The Greek Diet,
10. French Women don't get fat, Mireille Guiliano, Chatto and Windus, 2005, ISBN 0701178051
11. Natures medicines, Joel Swerdlow, National Geographic, 2000, ISBN 0792275861
12. Enquire within for everything – Houlston and Sons,1894
13. What the Doctors Don't Tell You, Lynne McTaggart, Harper Collins, 1996, ISBN 0722530242

Appendix 3. List of Books by the Author

This is a summary of books by Dick Handscombe written alone or jointly with his wife Clodagh. Those currently in print are marked*. New or second hand copies of the others are normally available on Amazon. Those authored as Richard rather than Dick are marked**.

Authentic Valencian Paellas - Self published - 2013**

Having a Great Retirement - Self published - 2013**

Making Waterless Gardens - Self published 2012**

Living Well From Our Garden - Self published - 2011**

Apartment Gardening Mediterranean Style – Santana Books April 2010* -Joint

Your garden in Spain – revised edition – Santana Books May 2007*- Joint

Growing healthy fruit in Spain – Santana Books – March 2007*- Joint

Growing healthy vegetables in Spain – Santana Books – December 2006*- Joint

Your Garden in Spain – Santana Books – 2005*- Joint

Practical Gardening on the Costa – Costa Blanca News –2002*- Jolint

Practical gardening on the Costa Blanca – Costa Blanca News – 2001*- Joint

Liderazgo estrategico – Los eslabones perdidos – McGraw Hill –1996**

El Jefe de producto – Guia practicas del Product Manager – McGraw Hill 1992**

Strategic Leadership – Managing the missing links – McGraw Hill 1993**

Strategic Leadership – The missing links – McGraw Hill 1989**

The product management handbook – McGraw Hill 1989**

Managing through people – ILO – 1985**

The Bankers management handbook – McGraw Hill 1978**

About the author Dick Handscombe

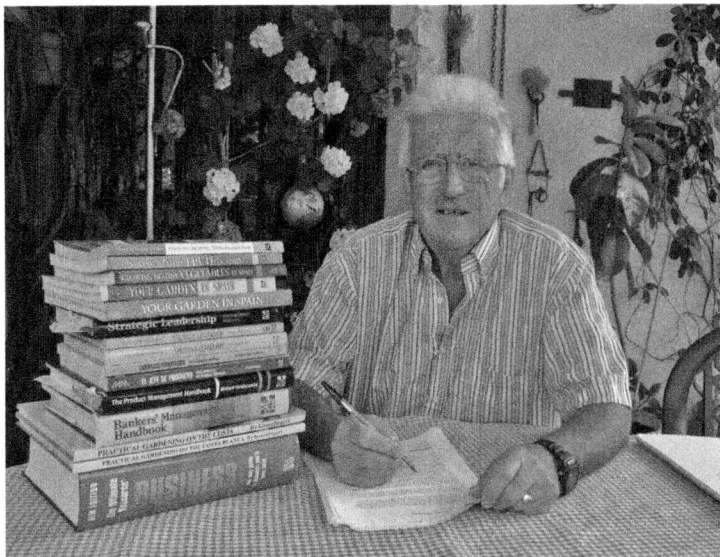

The following 12 points provide a factual background to the breadth and depth of the author's lifetime experience.

1. After two cancer operations in 1993 has lived retired in Spain. For previous five years the embryo mountainside garden was seen as a fitness camp. A place for physical mental and spiritual renewal away from a busy international work schedule.

2. Avoided chemo and radio therapy with support of surgeon by retiring early to a low stress valley in Spain which at the time was largely farmed and self sufficient. As the valley moved away from traditional natural artisan methods to chemical based agriculture a holistic self sufficient ecological garden was developed together with his wife Clodagh. Now 76 had started to garden largely ecologically since the age of five when he had is own small plot in wartime west London.

4. Has had 18 books published including this book. Eleven alone and seven with his wife Clodagh. See appendix 3 for full list.

5. Wholesome food from self produced produce, an holistic Mediterranean diet, regular mountain walking, fishing, writing and an attempt to paint ensure an active balanced retirement life.

6. Regular writer of articles for magazines, newspapers and websites, Own website is www.gardenspain. com. Has had several series of radio spots and appeared on a number of television programmes.

7. Widely travelled for work, research and pleasure. Worked in 30 countries and has lectured to and coached persons from more than a hundred countries. Has researched and holidayed in further counties from one side of the world to another.

8. Enjoys cooking, especially Spanish style, using the diversity of fresh home grown produce available daily.

9. Schooled at Haberdasher's Askes and graduated from University College London. An honorary professor of St. Thomas University Bolivia. Past Industrial Fellow of European Business School.

10. Worked in a wide range of industries and conscious of the pluses and minuses of their working practices and environment from the point of view of the wellness of employees, suppliers, trade customers, end users and eaters.

11. Member of the Mediterranean Garden Society, Slow Food, Fundem and Avinenca.

12. Contact via www.gardeninginspain.com or handscombe2@hotmail.com

Personal Notes

Personal Notes

CPSIA information can be obtained
at www.ICGtesting.com
Printed in the USA
LVOW03s2001061116
511850LV00008B/266/P